Lichen Sclerosus

Risk Factors of Lichen Sclerosus

By

Diogo Lincoln

Copyright@2023

Table of Contents

CHAPTER 1
Definition of Lichen Sclerosus

Lichen Sclerosus is a chronic, inflammatory skin condition that primarily affects the genital and anogenital areas. It is characterized by the presence of white, patchy skin that is often thin, fragile, and prone to itching and discomfort. Lichen Sclerosus can occur in both males and females, but it is more commonly diagnosed in women, especially postmenopausal women. The exact cause of Lichen Sclerosus is not fully understood, but it is believed to involve a combination of genetic, autoimmune, and hormonal factors.

The characteristic symptoms of Lichen Sclerosus include intense itching, pain, and discomfort in the affected areas. The skin may appear pale or white, and it can become thin and wrinkled over time. In severe cases, scarring and atrophy of the affected tissues can occur. Lichen Sclerosus can also extend beyond the genital region, affecting nearby areas such as the perianal region, inner thighs, and lower abdomen.

Lichen Sclerosus is a chronic condition with no known cure, but various treatment options are available to manage symptoms and prevent complications. Topical corticosteroids, such as clobetasol propionate, are commonly prescribed to reduce inflammation and alleviate symptoms. Calcineurin inhibitors, retinoids, and other immunomodulatory medications may also be used in certain cases.

In addition to medical treatments, self-care measures can play a crucial role in managing Lichen Sclerosus. These include practicing good hygiene, avoiding irritants, maintaining skin moisture with the use of moisturizers and emollients, and wearing loose-fitting clothing to minimize friction and irritation. Regular follow-up appointments with a healthcare provider are important to monitor the condition, assess treatment effectiveness, and address any concerns.

While Lichen Sclerosus is not a sexually transmitted infection, it can affect sexual function and intimacy due to pain, discomfort, and scarring. Psychological support and counseling may be beneficial for individuals experiencing emotional distress or body image concerns related to Lichen Sclerosus.

It is important to note that Lichen Sclerosus is a chronic condition that requires ongoing management. Early diagnosis and appropriate treatment can help alleviate symptoms, prevent complications, and improve quality of life. If you suspect you may have Lichen Sclerosus or are experiencing symptoms related to the condition, it is recommended to consult with a healthcare professional for an accurate diagnosis and personalized treatment plan.

CHAPTER 2

Treatment Options

Topical Corticosteroids

Topical corticosteroids are the most commonly prescribed and effective treatment for lichen sclerosus. These medications work by reducing inflammation, suppressing the immune response, and alleviating symptoms

Mechanism of action: Topical corticosteroids exert their therapeutic effects by binding to specific receptors in the cells, modulating gene expression, and inhibiting the production of inflammatory mediators. They have potent anti-inflammatory properties and help reduce the inflammation associated with Lichen Sclerosus.

Potency and formulations: Topical corticosteroids are available in various potencies, ranging from mild to high. The choice of potency depends on the severity and location of Lichen Sclerosus lesions. Mild corticosteroids (e.g., hydrocortisone) are often suitable for mild Lichen Sclerosus or sensitive areas, while more potent corticosteroids (e.g., clobetasol) may be necessary for moderate to severe Lichen Sclerosus or thickened skin.

These medications come in different formulations, including creams, ointments, lotions, and foams. Creams are generally preferred for acute or oozing lesions, while ointments provide better occlusion and hydration for chronic or dry lesions. The choice of formulation depends on individual preferences, lesion characteristics, and treatment response.

Application and duration: Topical corticosteroids should be applied directly to the affected areas of the skin as prescribed by a healthcare professional. The frequency and duration of application may vary depending on the severity of Lichen Sclerosus and the specific corticosteroid used. Initially, a higher potency corticosteroid may be prescribed for a few weeks to achieve disease control. Once symptoms improve, the frequency and strength of the medication are gradually tapered to the lowest effective dose for maintenance.

Treatment response: The response to topical corticosteroids can vary among individuals with Lichen Sclerosus. Some may experience significant improvement in symptoms, while others may have a partial response. It is important to have realistic expectations, as complete resolution of Lichen Sclerosus may not always be achievable. Regular follow-up with a healthcare professional is necessary to assess treatment response, adjust medication strength, and monitor for potential side effects.

Adverse effects: Topical corticosteroids, especially when used over a prolonged period or in high potency, can have potential side effects. These may include skin thinning, skin fragility, telangiectasia (visible blood vessels), striae (stretch marks), and temporary skin discoloration. It is crucial to use topical corticosteroids as directed and under the supervision of a healthcare professional to minimize the risk of side effects.

To minimize side effects, healthcare professionals may recommend using the "weekend" or "weekend plus one" regimen, where the medication is applied on specific days of the week to provide intermittent treatment and reduce exposure to corticosteroids.

Alternative formulations: In cases where corticosteroids are not well-tolerated or contraindicated, alternative formulations such as topical calcineurin inhibitors or retinoids may be considered (discussed in subsequent sections). These medications have different mechanisms of action and can be used as alternatives or in combination with topical corticosteroids.

Overall, topical corticosteroids play a pivotal role in the treatment of Lichen Sclerosus by reducing inflammation, controlling symptoms, and improving the quality of life for individuals with the condition. Proper application techniques, adherence to treatment plans, and regular follow-up care are essential for optimizing treatment outcomes and minimizing potential side effects.

Calcineurin Inhibitors

Calcineurin inhibitors are a class of topical medications that can be used as an alternative or adjunct to corticosteroids in the treatment of lichen sclerosus. These medications work by suppressing the immune response and reducing inflammation.

Mechanism of action: Calcineurin inhibitors, such as tacrolimus and pimecrolimus, inhibit calcineurin, an enzyme involved in the activation of T-lymphocytes. By inhibiting calcineurin, these medications help reduce the immune response and inflammation associated with Lichen Sclerosus.

Potency and formulations: Calcineurin inhibitors are available in various potencies, with tacrolimus being the stronger of the two. They are typically available as ointments and are suitable for application to sensitive areas or areas where corticosteroids may be less desirable, such as the face or thin skin. The choice of calcineurin inhibitor and formulation depends on the severity of Lichen Sclerosus, individual preferences, and treatment response.

Application and duration: Calcineurin inhibitors should be applied directly to the affected areas as prescribed by a healthcare professional. The frequency and duration of application may vary depending on the severity of Lichen Sclerosus and the specific medication used. Initially, a higher potency calcineurin inhibitor may be prescribed for a few weeks to achieve disease control. Once symptoms improve, the frequency and strength of the medication are gradually tapered to the lowest effective dose for maintenance.

Treatment response: The response to calcineurin inhibitors

can vary among individuals with Lichen Sclerosus. These medications may be particularly beneficial for individuals who are unable to tolerate or have poor response to corticosteroids. Some individuals may experience significant improvement in symptoms, while others may have a partial response. Regular follow-up with a healthcare professional is necessary to assess treatment response, adjust medication strength, and monitor for potential side effects.

Adverse effects: Calcineurin inhibitors are generally well-tolerated when used as directed. However, they can occasionally cause mild and transient side effects, such as burning, stinging, or itching at the application site. These side effects typically resolve with continued use. In rare cases, long-term use of calcineurin inhibitors may be associated with a slightly increased risk of skin infections or skin cancer, although the risk appears to be low.

Alternative or combination therapy: Calcineurin inhibitors can be used as alternatives or in combination with topical corticosteroids. In cases where corticosteroids are not well-tolerated or contraindicated, calcineurin inhibitors may provide an effective treatment option. They can also be used in a sequential or rotational manner with corticosteroids to minimize side effects and maintain disease control.

It is important to note that calcineurin inhibitors are generally considered second-line therapy for Lichen Sclerosus and are often reserved for cases where corticosteroids are not suitable or have not provided adequate symptom relief. The use of calcineurin inhibitors should be discussed with a healthcare professional who can evaluate individual circumstances, provide appropriate guidance, and closely monitor treatment response.

Retinoids

Retinoids, specifically topical tretinoin, are another treatment option for lichen sclerosus. Retinoids are derived from vitamin A and have been used in various dermatological conditions due to their anti-inflammatory and cell-regulating properties.

Mechanism of action: Retinoids modulate gene expression, promote cell differentiation, and have anti-inflammatory effects. In Lichen Sclerosus, topical tretinoin is believed to help normalize the differentiation and maturation of skin cells, reduce inflammation, and improve the structural integrity of the affected skin.

Application and duration: Topical tretinoin are usually applied directly to the affected areas of the skin as prescribed by a healthcare professional. The frequency and duration of application may vary depending on the severity of Lichen Sclerosus and individual response. It is important to follow the recommended treatment regimen and gradually increase the frequency of application to minimize potential skin irritation.

Treatment response: The response to retinoids can vary

among individuals with Lichen Sclerosus. Some may experience significant improvement in symptoms, while others may have a partial response. It is important to have realistic expectations, as complete resolution of Lichen Sclerosus may not always be achievable. Regular follow-up with a healthcare professional is necessary to assess treatment response, adjust medication strength, and monitor for potential side effects.

Adverse effects: Retinoids can cause skin irritation, dryness, redness, and increased sensitivity to sunlight. These side effects are usually mild and transient, and the skin gradually adapts to the medication with continued use. To minimize irritation, healthcare professionals may recommend starting with a lower concentration of tretinoin and gradually increasing the strength as tolerated.

Combination therapy: Retinoids can be used as part of a combination therapy approach for Lichen Sclerosus. They can be used in conjunction with corticosteroids or calcineurin inhibitors to enhance treatment response and address specific aspects of the disease, such as inflammation, cell proliferation, or skin barrier function. The use of combination therapy should be discussed with a healthcare professional who can evaluate individual circumstances and provide appropriate guidance.

It is important to note that retinoids, particularly tretinoin, are considered an off-label treatment for Lichen Sclerosus. This means that while they may be used by healthcare professionals based on their clinical judgment and experience, they are not specifically approved by regulatory authorities for the treatment of Lichen Sclerosus. The use of retinoids in Lichen Sclerosus should be discussed with a healthcare professional who can assess individual circumstances, provide appropriate guidance, and closely monitor treatment response.

Overall, topical corticosteroids, calcineurin inhibitors, and retinoids are important treatment options for lichen sclerosus. The choice of medication depends on individual factors such as the severity of Lichen Sclerosus, treatment response, preferences, and potential contraindications or side effects. Healthcare professionals can guide individuals with Lichen Sclerosus in selecting the most suitable treatment regimen and provide ongoing monitoring and support to optimize treatment outcomes.

Symptom Relief Measures

In addition to medical treatments, there are several symptom relief measures that can help manage the discomfort and improve the quality of life for individuals with lichen sclerosus. These measures aim to alleviate symptoms and promote overall well-being.

Hygiene practices: Maintaining proper hygiene is crucial in managing Lichen Sclerosus symptoms and preventing secondary infections. The following hygiene practices are recommended:

- Gentle cleansing: Use mild, fragrance-free cleansers or emollient washes to cleanse the affected areas. Avoid harsh soaps, perfumed products, or excessive scrubbing, as these can irritate the sensitive skin.

- Pat-drying: After cleansing, gently pat-dry the skin with a soft towel or air-dry to avoid friction or irritation.

- Avoid irritants: Avoid using products that contain potential irritants, such as dyes, perfumes, or harsh chemicals. Choose hypoallergenic or fragrance-free products whenever possible.

- Loose-fitting clothing: for loose-fitting, breathable clothing made from natural fibers (e.g., cotton) to minimize friction and allow air circulation. Avoid tight-fitting undergarments or clothing that may cause further irritation.

- Avoid scratching: Resist the urge to scratch or rub the affected areas, as this can worsen the symptoms and potentially lead to skin damage or infection. If itching is severe, healthcare professionals may recommend topical or oral antihistamines to help alleviate the itchiness.

Moisturizers and emollients: Regular use of moisturizers and emollients can help hydrate and protect the affected skin in Lichen Sclerosus. These products help maintain the skin barrier function and reduce dryness, itchiness, and discomfort. Here are some recommendations for moisturizer use:

- Choose appropriate products: for fragrance-free, hypoallergenic moisturizers or emollients that are specifically formulated for sensitive skin. Avoid products that contain potential irritants, such as alcohol or fragrances.

- Application technique: Apply moisturizers or emollients to the affected areas after cleansing and gently pat-drying the skin. Use a gentle, upward motion to spread the product evenly. It is recommended to apply moisturizers at least twice daily or as needed to maintain skin hydration.

- Ointments vs. creams: Ointments are generally more occlusive and provide

better hydration and
protection for dry or
cracked skin. Creams or
lotions may be suitable for
less severe or acute Lichen
Sclerosus lesions. The
choice of formulation
depends on individual
preferences, lesion
characteristics, and
treatment response.

- Combination with medical
  treatments: Moisturizers
  and emollients can be used
  in combination with
  medical treatments, such as
  topical corticosteroids or
  calcineurin inhibitors, to
  enhance treatment

outcomes and provide additional symptom relief.

Warm baths or sitz baths: Taking warm baths or sitz baths can provide temporary relief from itching, discomfort, and inflammation associated with Lichen Sclerosus. Here are some guidelines for bath therapy:

- Warm water: Fill the bathtub or sitz bath with warm water at a comfortable temperature. Avoid using hot water, as it can further irritate the skin.

- Duration: Soak in the bath for 10-15 minutes to allow the water to soothe the affected areas. Gentle movement or stirring the water with your hand can help distribute the soothing effects.

- Drying: After the bath, gently pat-dry the skin with a soft towel. Avoid rubbing or harsh towel-drying, as it can cause further irritation.

- Moisturize: Apply a moisturizer or emollient immediately after the bath to seal in the moisture and hydrate the skin.

Topical barrier creams or ointments: Barrier creams or ointments can provide an additional protective layer on the affected skin, reducing friction and irritation. These products help create a barrier between the skin and potential irritants. Here are some considerations for using topical barrier creams or ointments:

- Ingredients: Look for products that contain ingredients such as dimethicone, zinc oxide, or petrolatum, which form a protective barrier on the skin.

- Application: Apply a thin layer of the barrier cream or ointment to the affected areas after cleansing and drying the skin. Reapply as needed or as directed by a healthcare professional.

- Combination with other treatments: Topical barrier creams or ointments can be used in combination with medical treatments to enhance their efficacy and provide additional protection for the skin.

Pain relief measures: Lichen Sclerosus can sometimes cause pain or discomfort, especially during intercourse or urination. The following measures can help alleviate pain:

- Lubricants: Use water-based lubricants during sexual intercourse to reduce friction and discomfort. Avoid products that contain potential irritants, such as fragrances or dyes.

- Topical anesthetics: In some cases, healthcare professionals may recommend the use of topical anesthetics, such as lidocaine gel, to numb the affected areas temporarily and reduce pain or discomfort.

- Urination techniques: For individuals experiencing pain during urination, strategies such as sitting in a warm bath or using a peri-bottle filled with warm water can help alleviate discomfort.

Psychological support: Living with Lichen Sclerosus can be emotionally challenging for some individuals due to the chronic nature of the condition and its impact on sexual function and body image. Seeking psychological support, such as counseling or support groups, can provide valuable emotional support, coping strategies, and a sense of community. These resources can help individuals better manage the psychological aspects of Lichen Sclerosus and improve overall well-being.

It is important to remember that symptom relief measures are supportive measures that can help manage Lichen Sclerosus symptoms but may not address the underlying disease process. They should be used in conjunction with medical treatments and under the guidance of a healthcare professional. Regular follow-up care is crucial to monitor treatment response, adjust management strategies, and ensure overall disease control.

Surgical Interventions

In certain cases of lichen sclerosus, surgical interventions may be considered to address specific complications or improve symptoms. Surgical options for Lichen Sclerosus aim to alleviate anatomical changes, correct functional impairments, or manage severe disease that is unresponsive to medical treatments. Here is a detailed overview of surgical interventions for Lichen Sclerosus:

Preputioplasty or circumcision: In males with Lichen Sclerosus, preputioplasty or circumcision may be recommended to address phimosis (inability to retract the foreskin) and relieve symptoms. Preputioplasty involves preserving the foreskin by making incisions and sutures to

widen the preputial opening,
allowing for improved hygiene
and reduced constriction.
Circumcision involves the
complete removal of the foreskin
and is sometimes recommended
for severe or recurrent cases of
Lichen Sclerosus.

Vulvar reconstruction or
labiaplasty: In females with
Lichen Sclerosus, vulvar
reconstruction or labiaplasty may
be considered to address severe
scarring, fusion, or anatomical
changes that significantly impact
daily activities or sexual
function. These procedures
involve reshaping or
reconstructing the vulvar area to
alleviate symptoms, improve

appearance, and restore functionality.

Dilatation or vaginal surgery: In some cases of Lichen Sclerosus, vaginal involvement can cause narrowing, fusion, or scarring, leading to pain during intercourse or difficulty with sexual activity. Vaginal dilatation, performed under the guidance of a healthcare professional, involves using progressively larger dilators to stretch and expand the vaginal opening and canal. Vaginal surgery, such as vaginoplasty or vaginectomy, may be considered in severe cases to address significant vaginal narrowing, scarring, or obstruction.

Other surgical interventions: In rare cases, surgical interventions such as skin grafting or plastic surgery may be necessary to manage severe Lichen Sclerosus related complications or disfigurement. These procedures involve the transplantation of healthy skin or reconstruction techniques to improve function, appearance, or quality of life.

It is important to note that surgical interventions are typically reserved for individuals with Lichen Sclerosus who have failed to respond to conservative treatments or who have significant functional or anatomical impairments. The decision to undergo surgery should be made in consultation with a healthcare professional experienced in the management of Lichen Sclerosus. They will assess the individual's specific circumstances, treatment response, and potential risks and benefits associated with the surgical intervention.

Surgical interventions for Lichen Sclerosus should be performed by qualified healthcare professionals, such as gynecologists, urologists, or plastic surgeons, who have expertise in managing Lichen Sclerosus complications. Regular follow-up care and close monitoring after surgery are essential to ensure proper healing, manage potential complications, and optimize treatment outcomes.

It is important to emphasize that while surgical interventions can provide significant relief and improve quality of life for individuals with Lichen Sclerosus, they do not cure the underlying disease. Lichen Sclerosus is a chronic condition that requires ongoing management and monitoring even after surgical intervention. Combining surgical interventions with appropriate medical treatments and lifestyle modifications is key to achieving long-term disease control and minimizing the risk of recurrence or complications.

symptom relief measures such as hygiene practices, moisturizers and emollients, warm baths or sitz baths, topical barrier creams or ointments, pain relief measures, and psychological support can help alleviate discomfort and improve the quality of life for individuals with lichen sclerosus. Surgical interventions, including preputioplasty or circumcision, vulvar reconstruction or labiaplasty, dilatation or vaginal surgery, and other procedures, may be considered in cases where conservative treatments have been ineffective or significant functional or anatomical impairments are present. The decision to pursue surgical intervention should be made in consultation with a healthcare professional who can evaluate individual circumstances, provide appropriate guidance, and ensure comprehensive care.

CHAPTER 3

Psychological Well-being

Sexual Relationships and Intimacy

Lichen sclerosus can have a significant impact on sexual relationships and intimacy. The symptoms and physical discomfort associated with Lichen Sclerosus can affect sexual function, desire, and overall sexual well-being. we delve into the impact of Lichen Sclerosus on sexual relationships and intimacy, as well as coping strategies and support for individuals and couples facing these challenges.

1. Painful Intercourse: One of the primary concerns for individuals with Lichen Sclerosus is painful intercourse, known as dyspareunia. The inflammation, scarring, and atrophy associated with Lichen Sclerosus can cause discomfort, burning sensations, and tearing during sexual activity. This can lead to anxiety, avoidance of sexual encounters, and strain in relationships.

2. Decreased Sexual Desire: Lichen Sclerosus can also lead to a decrease in sexual desire or libido. The physical discomfort and emotional distress associated with the condition can diminish interest in sexual activities. Individuals may experience a loss of sexual confidence and reduced self-esteem, further impacting their desire for intimacy.

3. Emotional and Psychological Impact: Lichen Sclerosus can have a profound emotional and psychological impact on individuals and their

partners. Feelings of frustration, sadness, and anxiety may arise due to the challenges faced in maintaining a fulfilling sexual relationship. The impact of Lichen Sclerosus on body image, self-esteem, and overall well-being can also contribute to difficulties in intimacy.

4. Relationship Strain: The challenges associated with Lichen Sclerosus can put strain on intimate relationships. Partners may feel frustrated, helpless, or worried about causing pain to their loved one. Miscommunication, lack of

understanding, and decreased intimacy can create tension and distance between partners.

Coping Strategies and Support:

1. Open Communication: Open and honest communication with one's partner is crucial when dealing with the impact of Lichen Sclerosus on sexual relationships. Sharing concerns, fears, and physical limitations can foster understanding, empathy, and support. Discussing and exploring alternative intimate activities that are

comfortable and
pleasurable can help
maintain a sense of
connection.

2. Education and Counseling:
Educating oneself and one's
partner about Lichen
Sclerosus and its impact on
sexual well-being can
facilitate understanding and
empathy. Couples may
consider seeking
counseling or therapy from
professionals experienced
in addressing sexual health
and relationship issues. Sex
therapy can provide
guidance on
communication, techniques
for managing pain, and

strategies to enhance
intimacy.

3. Experimentation and
   Adaptation: Exploring
   different sexual activities
   and finding alternative
   ways to express intimacy
   can help maintain a
   fulfilling and satisfying
   sexual relationship.
   Experimenting with
   different positions,
   lubricants, and aids can
   alleviate discomfort and
   enhance pleasure. Open-
   mindedness, creativity, and
   a willingness to adapt can
   play a crucial role in
   overcoming challenges.

4. Psychological Support: Seeking support from mental health professionals, such as therapists or counselors, can assist individuals and couples in navigating the emotional impact of Lichen Sclerosus on sexual relationships. Counseling can provide a safe space to address concerns, manage anxiety or depression, and develop coping strategies to enhance overall well-being.

5. Support Groups: Joining support groups specific to Lichen Sclerosus or sexual health can be invaluable for individuals and couples

facing similar challenges. Engaging with others who have firsthand experience with Lichen Sclerosus can provide a sense of validation, encouragement, and practical advice for managing the impact on sexual relationships and intimacy.

6. Self-Care and Self-Exploration: Engaging in self-care practices that promote self-acceptance, self-compassion, and self-exploration can contribute to improved sexual well-being. This may involve practices such as mindfulness, self-pleasure,

self-affirmation, and self-education about one's own body and sexual desires.

7. Professional Guidance: Consulting with healthcare professionals specializing in sexual health, such as gynecologists, urologists, or sexual medicine specialists, can provide tailored medical interventions and guidance specific to Lichen Sclerosus related sexual issues. They can recommend appropriate treatments, medications, or therapies that may alleviate symptoms and enhance sexual function.

It is essential to approach the impact of Lichen Sclerosus on sexual relationships and intimacy with patience, compassion, and a willingness to adapt. Every individual and couple's experience is unique, and finding the right strategies and support may require trial and error. Seeking professional help, maintaining open communication, and prioritizing emotional well-being can contribute to nurturing healthy and satisfying sexual relationships in the context of Lichen Sclerosus.

CHAPTER 4

Etiology and Risk Factors of Lichen Sclerosus

Lichen sclerosus is a chronic inflammatory skin condition that primarily affects the genital and anogenital areas. While the exact cause of remains unknown, several factors are believed to contribute to its development. Here are the potential etiological factors and risk factors associated with Lichen Sclerosus.

Etiology:

1. Autoimmune Dysfunction: Lichen Sclerosus is considered to have an autoimmune component, as the immune system plays a role in the pathogenesis of the condition. Autoimmune diseases occur when the immune system mistakenly attacks healthy tissues in the body. In Lichen Sclerosus, it is thought that immune dysfunction leads to an inflammatory response, resulting in the characteristic symptoms and changes in the affected areas.

2. Genetic Predisposition: Genetic factors may contribute to the development of Lichen Sclerosus. Studies have shown that individuals with a family history of Lichen Sclerosus are more likely to develop the condition themselves. However, specific genetic markers or mutations associated with Lichen Sclerosus have not yet been identified.

3. Hormonal Imbalance: Hormonal imbalances, particularly in postmenopausal women, have been implicated in the development of Lichen

Sclerosus. The decline in estrogen levels during menopause may contribute to the thinning and atrophy of the genital skin, making it more susceptible to inflammation and damage. However, Lichen Sclerosus can also occur in prepubertal girls and men, suggesting that hormonal factors alone do not account for all cases.

4. Infectious Agents: Some research suggests a potential link between Lichen Sclerosus and certain infectious agents, such as the human papillomavirus (HPV) and

Borrelia burgdorferi, the bacterium responsible for Lyme disease. However, the role of these agents in Lichen Sclerosus development is still unclear, and further research is needed to establish a definitive connection.

Risk Factors:

1. Age and Gender: Lichen Sclerosus can affect individuals of any age and gender. However, certain age groups and genders are more susceptible. In females, Lichen Sclerosus commonly affects

postmenopausal women, although it can also occur in prepubertal girls. In males, Lichen Sclerosus typically occurs in adulthood. The reason for the gender disparity is not fully understood, but hormonal differences and genetic factors may contribute.

2. Genetic Factors: As mentioned earlier, having a family history of Lichen Sclerosus increases the risk of developing the condition. The specific genes or genetic variants involved in Lichen Sclerosus susceptibility

have not yet been identified, highlighting the need for further research in this area.

3. Personal History of Autoimmune Diseases: Individuals with a personal history of autoimmune diseases, such as thyroid disorders, vitiligo, or alopecia areata, may have an increased risk of developing Lichen Sclerosus. The shared immune dysregulation underlying these conditions may contribute to the development of Lichen Sclerosus.

4. Trauma or Injury: Trauma or injury to the affected areas, such as previous surgery, chronic irritation, or repeated rubbing, may increase the risk of developing Lichen Sclerosus. It is thought that tissue damage and subsequent inflammation can trigger the immune response seen in Lichen Sclerosus.

5. Chronic Inflammation: Chronic inflammation in the affected areas may be a risk factor for Lichen Sclerosus. Conditions associated with chronic inflammation, such as

chronic infections, chronic irritation, or autoimmune diseases, may increase the likelihood of Lichen Sclerosus development. The underlying inflammatory processes may contribute to the progression of Lichen Sclerosus and its associated symptoms.

6. Personal Hygiene Practices: While not definitively established, poor personal hygiene practices have been suggested as potential risk factors for Lichen Sclerosus. Excessive cleansing, use of harsh soaps, and inadequate

drying of the genital area may disrupt the delicate balance of the skin, making it more susceptible to inflammation and damage. However, the role of hygiene practices in Lichen Sclerosus development is still a subject of debate and requires further investigation.

It is important to note that while these factors are believed to contribute to the development of Lichen Sclerosus, they do not guarantee the development of the condition. Many individuals with one or more risk factors may never develop Lichen Sclerosus, while others without any apparent risk factors may develop the condition. The complex interplay between genetic predisposition, hormonal factors, immune dysfunction, and environmental triggers is still not fully understood and requires ongoing research.

The etiology of Lichen Sclerosus is multifactorial, with autoimmune dysfunction, genetic predisposition, hormonal imbalances, infectious agents, and chronic inflammation being proposed as potential contributors. Understanding these factors can help in the identification of individuals at higher risk and the development of targeted preventive strategies

and treatment approaches.
Further research is needed to
unravel the precise mechanisms
underlying Lichen Sclerosus
development and to improve our
ability to prevent and manage
this challenging condition.

CHAPTER 5

Pathophysiology of Lichen Sclerosus

Immune System Involvement

Lichen Sclerosus is a chronic inflammatory skin condition that primarily affects the genital and anogenital areas. The precise pathophysiology of Lichen Sclerosus is not fully understood, but growing evidence suggests that immune system dysfunction plays a significant role in its development and progression.

The immune system is responsible for defending the body against foreign invaders, such as bacteria, viruses, and other pathogens. In Lichen Sclerosus, it is believed that an abnormal immune response leads to chronic inflammation, tissue damage, and the characteristic symptoms observed in affected individuals. The immune system's involvement in the pathophysiology of Lichen Sclerosus:

1. Autoimmunity: Lichen Sclerosus is considered to have an autoimmune component, meaning that the immune system mistakenly targets and

attacks healthy tissues in the body. Autoimmune diseases occur when the immune system loses its ability to distinguish between self and non-self, leading to an attack on the body's own tissues. In Lichen Sclerosus, the immune system targets the skin in the affected areas, triggering an inflammatory response.

2. T-cell Mediated Immune Response: T-cells, a type of white blood cell, play a crucial role in the immune response. Studies have shown that Lichen Sclerosus is characterized

by an accumulation of T-cells in the affected skin. These T-cells, particularly CD8+ cytotoxic T-cells, infiltrate the skin and release pro-inflammatory cytokines, such as interferon-gamma (IFN-γ) and tumor necrosis factor-alpha (TNF-α). These cytokines promote inflammation and tissue damage, contributing to the pathogenesis of Lichen Sclerosus.

3. Inflammatory Cascade: The chronic inflammation observed in Lichen Sclerosus is thought to result from an imbalance in

the production of pro-inflammatory and anti-inflammatory factors. In addition to T-cells, other immune cells, such as mast cells and macrophages, are also involved in the inflammatory cascade seen in Lichen Sclerosus. Mast cells release histamine and other inflammatory mediators, while macrophages contribute to tissue damage by producing reactive oxygen species and proteases.

4. Cytokine Imbalance: Cytokines, small proteins produced by immune cells, play a critical role in

immune regulation and the communication between cells. In Lichen Sclerosus, there is an altered cytokine profile in the affected skin. Pro-inflammatory cytokines, such as IFN-γ and TNF-α, are upregulated, while anti-inflammatory cytokines, such as interleukin-10 (IL-10) and transforming growth factor-beta (TGF-β), are downregulated. This imbalance perpetuates the inflammatory response, leading to tissue destruction and symptoms associated with Lichen Sclerosus.

5. Altered Extracellular Matrix: The extracellular matrix (ECM) provides structural support to tissues and plays a role in wound healing and tissue remodeling. In Lichen Sclerosus, there are changes in the ECM composition, characterized by an increase in collagen deposition and elastin degradation. These alterations in the ECM can lead to tissue atrophy, scarring, and loss of elasticity, further exacerbating the symptoms of Lichen Sclerosus.

6. Autoantibodies: Some
studies have reported the
presence of autoantibodies
in individuals with Lichen
Sclerosus. Autoantibodies
are antibodies that
mistakenly target and attack
the body's own tissues. The
significance of these
autoantibodies in Lichen
Sclerosus pathophysiology
is still under investigation,
and their exact role in
disease development and
progression remains
unclear.

It is important to note that while
immune system involvement is a
prominent feature in Lichen
Sclerosus, the exact triggers and

mechanisms that initiate and perpetuate the immune response are yet to be fully understood. Additionally, the immune system's contribution to Lichen Sclerosus may vary among individuals, and further research is needed to elucidate the complex interplay between immune dysfunction, genetic predisposition, and environmental factors in the pathophysiology of Lichen Sclerosus.

Lichen Sclerosus is characterized by immune system dysregulation, including an autoimmune component, T-cell-mediated immune response, inflammatory cascade, cytokine imbalance, altered ECM, and potential involvement of autoantibodies. Understanding the immune system's role in Lichen Sclerosus pathophysiology is crucial for the development of targeted therapeutic approaches aimed at modulating the immune response and alleviating the symptoms associated with this chronic condition.

Autoimmune Mechanisms

Lichen Sclerosus is a chronic inflammatory skin condition that primarily affects the genital and anogenital areas. While the exact cause of Lichen Sclerosus remains unclear, there is growing evidence to suggest an autoimmune component in its pathophysiology. Autoimmunity refers to a condition where the immune system mistakenly targets and attacks the body's own tissues. In Lichen Sclerosus, the immune system specifically targets the skin in the affected areas, leading to inflammation and tissue damage. These are autoimmune mechanisms believed to be involved in Lichen Sclerosus:

1. Loss of Immune Tolerance: Immune tolerance is the normal state in which the immune system recognizes and tolerates the body's own tissues, preventing an

immune response against self-antigens. In Lichen Sclerosus, there appears to be a breakdown in immune tolerance, resulting in an immune response against self-antigens in the skin. This loss of immune tolerance may be due to various factors, including genetic predisposition, environmental triggers, and dysregulation of immune checkpoints.

2. Autoantibodies: Autoantibodies are antibodies that target and attack the body's own tissues. In Lichen Sclerosus, autoantibodies

have been detected in some individuals, suggesting an autoimmune response. These autoantibodies may target specific proteins or structures within the skin, leading to inflammation and tissue damage. The presence of autoantibodies in Lichen Sclerosus supports the hypothesis of an autoimmune component in its pathophysiology, although the specific targets and their significance are still under investigation.

3. T-Cell Dysregulation: T-cells are a type of white blood cell that play a crucial role in the immune

response. In Lichen Sclerosus, there is evidence of T-cell dysregulation, particularly an increase in CD4+ and CD8+ T-cells in the affected skin. CD4+ T-cells are involved in orchestrating immune responses, while CD8+ T-cells have cytotoxic properties. The accumulation of these T-cells suggests an ongoing immune response and inflammation in the affected areas. These activated T-cells release pro-inflammatory cytokines, such as interferon-gamma (IFN-γ)

and tumor necrosis factor-alpha (TNF-α), which further contribute to tissue damage and inflammation.

4. Dendritic Cell Dysfunction: Dendritic cells are antigen-presenting cells that play a critical role in initiating and regulating immune responses. In Lichen Sclerosus, there is evidence of dendritic cell dysfunction, which may contribute to the abnormal immune response observed in the condition. Dysfunctional dendritic cells may fail to properly present self-antigens to T-cells, leading to a

breakdown in immune tolerance and the development of an autoimmune response.

5. Genetic Predisposition: Genetic factors have been implicated in the development of Lichen Sclerosus, suggesting a possible genetic predisposition to autoimmune mechanisms. Certain genetic variations may contribute to the dysregulation of the immune system, making individuals more susceptible to developing Lichen Sclerosus. However, the specific

genes and their exact role in Lichen Sclerosus pathophysiology have not been fully elucidated and require further investigation.

It is important to note that while autoimmune mechanisms appear to be involved in Lichen Sclerosus, the exact triggers and mechanisms that initiate and perpetuate the autoimmune response are not yet fully understood. Additionally, it is likely that autoimmune mechanisms interact with other factors, such as hormonal imbalances, environmental triggers, and infectious agents, to contribute to the development and progression of Lichen Sclerosus.

Lichen Sclerosus is believed to have an autoimmune component, involving loss of immune tolerance, the presence of autoantibodies, T-cell dysregulation, dendritic cell dysfunction, and potential genetic predisposition. These autoimmune mechanisms lead to chronic inflammation and tissue damage in the affected areas. Understanding the autoimmune aspects of Lichen Sclerosus is crucial for the development of targeted therapeutic approaches aimed at modulating the immune response and mitigating the symptoms associated with this complex condition.

Genetic Factors

Lichen Sclerosus is a chronic inflammatory skin condition that primarily affects the genital and anogenital areas. While the exact cause of Lichen Sclerosus is still not fully understood, genetic factors are believed to play a role in its development and progression. Genetic factors contribute to an individual's susceptibility to Lichen Sclerosus by influencing various aspects of the immune system, skin structure, and hormonal regulation. Here, are the genetic factors associated with Lichen Sclerosus:

1. Familial Clustering: Observations of Lichen Sclerosus cases within families suggest a potential genetic component in the development of the condition. There is evidence to support the familial clustering of Lichen Sclerosus, indicating a hereditary predisposition. Studies have shown an increased risk of Lichen Sclerosus among first-degree relatives of affected individuals, suggesting a genetic influence. However, the

specific genes involved and their inheritance patterns are yet to be fully elucidated.

2. Human Leukocyte Antigen (HLA) Associations: The human leukocyte antigen (HLA) system plays a critical role in immune regulation and the recognition of self and non-self-antigens. Genetic variations within the HLA region have been associated with Lichen Sclerosus susceptibility. Certain HLA alleles, such as HLA-DQ7 and HLA-DRB1*04, have been found to be more prevalent in individuals

with Lichen Sclerosus
compared to the general
population. These HLA
associations suggest an
involvement of immune
dysregulation in Lichen
Sclerosus pathophysiology.

3. Polymorphisms in Immune-
Related Genes:
Polymorphisms are
variations in DNA
sequences that can
influence gene function and
protein expression. Several
polymorphisms in immune-
related genes have been
implicated in Lichen
Sclerosus susceptibility.
For example, variations in
genes encoding cytokines,

such as tumor necrosis factor-alpha (TNF-α) and interleukin-10 (IL-10), have been associated with an increased risk of Lichen Sclerosus. These genetic variations may impact immune responses, leading to an altered inflammatory environment and tissue damage seen in Lichen Sclerosus.

4. Skin Barrier Genes: The skin acts as a physical barrier, protecting the body from environmental insults. Genetic variations in genes involved in skin barrier function have been proposed as potential

contributors to Lichen Sclerosus pathophysiology. For instance, mutations in filaggrin (FLG) gene, which encodes a protein important for maintaining the integrity of the skin barrier, have been associated with an increased risk of Lichen Sclerosus. Impaired skin barrier function may allow for the penetration of irritants and pathogens, triggering an abnormal immune response.

5. Hormonal Regulation: Hormonal factors, particularly estrogen, have been implicated in the

development and progression of Lichen Sclerosus. Estrogen receptors are present in the skin, and estrogen has been shown to influence immune responses and skin integrity. Genetic variations in genes involved in estrogen metabolism and receptor signaling pathways may influence an individual's hormonal balance and, consequently, their susceptibility to Lichen Sclerosus.

6. Epigenetic Modifications: Epigenetic modifications refer to changes in gene expression that do not

involve alterations in the underlying DNA sequence. These modifications can be influenced by various factors, including environmental exposures and lifestyle choices. Epigenetic changes have been proposed as potential contributors to Lichen Sclerosus development. DNA methylation, histone modifications, and microRNA dysregulation are examples of epigenetic mechanisms that may influence gene expression and immune responses in Lichen Sclerosus.

It is important to note that Lichen Sclerosus is a complex condition, and the contribution of genetic factors may vary among individuals. The interplay between genetic predisposition, immune dysregulation, environmental triggers, and other factors is not fully understood and requires further research.

Genetic factors contribute to an individual's susceptibility to Lichen Sclerosus. Familial clustering, HLA associations, polymorphisms in immune-related genes, skin barrier gene variations, hormonal regulation, and epigenetic modifications are all potential genetic factors involved in Lichen Sclerosus pathophysiology. Understanding the genetic underpinnings of Lichen Sclerosus can provide insights into the disease mechanisms and help identify individuals at higher risk, facilitating early detection and targeted interventions.

Skin Barrier Dysfunction

Lichen Sclerosus is a chronic inflammatory skin condition that primarily affects the genital and anogenital areas. While the exact cause of Lichen Sclerosus is not fully understood, skin barrier dysfunction has been proposed as one of the contributing factors in its pathophysiology. The skin barrier serves as the body's first line of defense, protecting against external pathogens, irritants, and maintaining optimal hydration. Disruption of the skin barrier can lead to increased susceptibility to inflammation and tissue damage. Here, are the role of skin barrier dysfunction in Lichen Sclerosus:

1. Epidermal Barrier Impairment: The epidermis is the outermost layer of the skin and plays a crucial role in maintaining the integrity of the skin barrier. In Lichen Sclerosus, there is evidence of epidermal barrier impairment, characterized by alterations in the structure and

function of the epidermal cells. Studies have shown reduced expression of key proteins involved in skin barrier function, such as filaggrin, loricrin, and involucrin, in the affected skin of Lichen Sclerosus patients. These changes compromise the skin's ability to retain moisture and provide protection against external insults.

2. Altered Lipid Composition: Lipids are essential components of the skin barrier, forming a protective barrier against water loss and preventing the entry of irritants and

microorganisms. In Lichen Sclerosus, there are alterations in the lipid composition of the affected skin. Specifically, there is a decrease in the levels of ceramides, cholesterol, and free fatty acids, which are crucial for maintaining an effective skin barrier. This lipid imbalance can lead to increased permeability of the skin, allowing for the penetration of irritants and triggering an inflammatory response.

3. Abnormalities in Tight Junction Proteins: Tight junctions are specialized structures that connect

adjacent epidermal cells, forming a physical barrier and regulating the passage of molecules between cells. In Lichen Sclerosus, there is evidence of abnormalities in tight junction proteins, such as claudin-1 and occludin. Disruption of tight junctions can compromise the integrity of the skin barrier, leading to increased permeability and inflammation.

4. Impaired Natural Moisturizing Factors (NMFs): NMFs are a group of water-soluble compounds naturally present in the stratum

corneum, the outermost layer of the epidermis. They play a crucial role in maintaining skin hydration and integrity. In Lichen Sclerosus, there is a reduction in the levels of NMFs, including urea, lactate, and amino acids, in the affected skin. This deficiency in NMFs can disrupt the water-holding capacity of the skin, contributing to dryness, cracking, and further barrier impairment.

5. Microbial Dysbiosis: The skin is home to a diverse microbial community known as the skin

microbiota. The microbiota plays a crucial role in maintaining skin health and barrier function. In Lichen Sclerosus, there is evidence of microbial dysbiosis, characterized by alterations in the composition and diversity of the skin microbiota. This dysbiosis can disrupt the delicate balance between commensal and pathogenic bacteria, further compromising the skin barrier and promoting inflammation.

It is important to note that skin barrier dysfunction in Lichen Sclerosus may be influenced by various factors, including genetic predisposition, immune dysregulation, hormonal imbalances, and environmental triggers. The interplay between these factors can exacerbate the skin barrier impairment and contribute to the chronic inflammatory response observed in Lichen Sclerosus.

Understanding the role of skin barrier dysfunction in Lichen Sclerosus pathophysiology is crucial for the development of targeted therapeutic approaches. Strategies aimed at restoring and strengthening the skin barrier, such as emollients and moisturizers, are commonly employed in the management of Lichen Sclerosus. These products help replenish moisture, repair the skin barrier, and alleviate symptoms such as dryness and itching. Emollients, which are lipid-based formulations, can help seal in moisture and restore the skin's natural lipid barrier. They provide a protective layer on the skin surface, reducing water loss and promoting hydration.

In addition to topical moisturizers, other treatment modalities that target skin barrier dysfunction in Lichen Sclerosus include:

1. Topical Corticosteroids: Topical corticosteroids are commonly prescribed in the treatment of Lichen Sclerosus. They work by reducing inflammation and suppressing the immune response in the affected area. By alleviating inflammation, corticosteroids can help restore the integrity of the skin barrier and improve symptoms. However, long-term use of potent corticosteroids should be monitored closely to

minimize potential side effects.

2. Calcineurin Inhibitors: Calcineurin inhibitors, such as tacrolimus and pimecrolimus, are immunomodulatory agents that inhibit T-cell activation and cytokine production. They are considered alternatives to corticosteroids, especially in sensitive areas or when corticosteroid use is not well-tolerated. Calcineurin inhibitors can help reduce inflammation and improve skin barrier function in Lichen Sclerosus.

3. Retinoids: Retinoids, derived from vitamin A, have been used in the treatment of Lichen Sclerosus due to their anti-inflammatory and immunomodulatory effects. They help regulate cell growth and differentiation, promoting the regeneration of healthy skin cells. Topical retinoids, such as tretinoin and isotretinoin, may be prescribed to improve the skin barrier function and reduce inflammation in Lichen Sclerosus.

4. Symptom Relief Measures: Along with medical

treatments, various self-care measures can help alleviate symptoms and support the skin barrier in Lichen Sclerosus. These include:

- Gentle cleansing: Use mild, fragrance-free cleansers and avoid harsh soaps or cleansing agents that can further irritate the skin.

- Avoid irritants: Identify and avoid potential irritants that can exacerbate symptoms, such as tight-fitting clothing,

synthetic fabrics, and
certain personal care
products.

- Moisturize regularly:
  Apply moisturizers or
  emollients to the
  affected areas
  multiple times a day
  to maintain skin
  hydration and support
  the skin barrier
  function.

- Avoid scratching:
  Scratching can
  worsen symptoms and
  damage the skin.
  Keep nails short and
  consider using
  protective measures,

such as wearing
gloves during sleep,
to prevent scratching
during the night.

- Cool compresses:
  Applying cool
  compresses or ice
  packs to the affected
  areas can help soothe
  itching and reduce
  inflammation.

Addressing skin barrier
dysfunction is an essential
component of Lichen Sclerosus
management. By restoring the
integrity of the skin barrier,
reducing inflammation, and
promoting skin hydration,

targeted treatment strategies aim to alleviate symptoms, prevent further damage, and improve the overall condition of the skin. It is important to work closely with a healthcare professional to determine the most suitable treatment plan based on individual needs and to monitor the response to treatment over time.

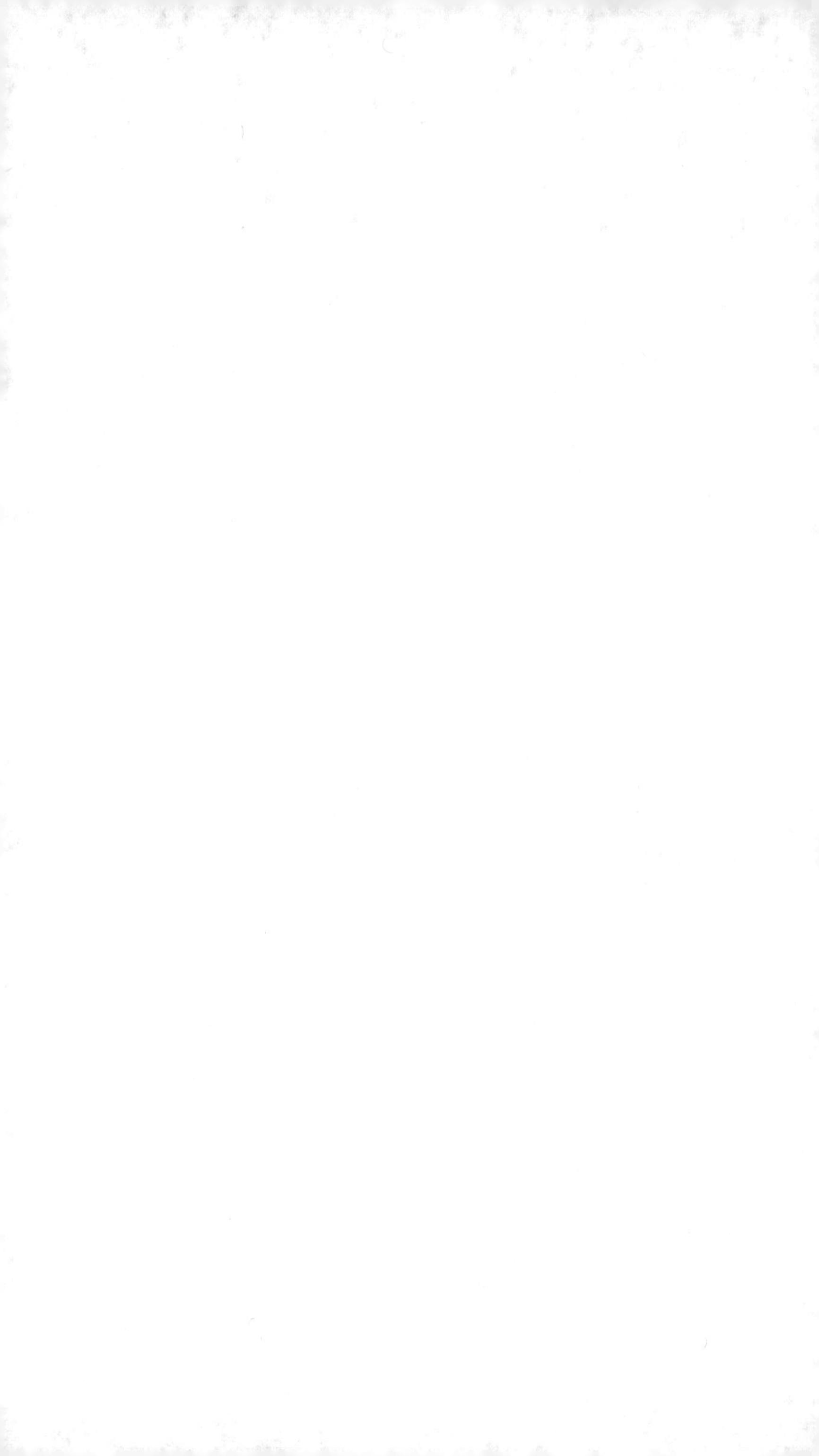

www.ingramcontent.com/pod-product-compliance
Lightning Source LLC
Chambersburg PA
CBHW051819250726
48659CB00005B/1562